My Air Fryer Lunch

A Handful of Quick, Delicious Recipes for
Your Air Fryer Meals

Dalia Gillespie

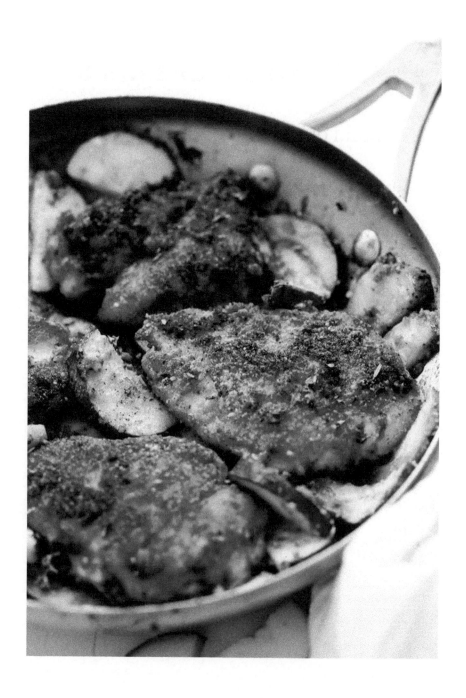

3

TABLE OF CONTENT

Asian Halibut

Preparation time: 30 minutes

Cooking time: 10 minutes

Servings: 3

Ingredients:

- 1 pound halibut steaks
- 2/3 cup soy sauce
- ¼ cup sugar
- 2 tablespoons lime juice
- ½ cup mirin
- ¼ teaspoon red pepper flakes, crushed
- ¼ cup orange juice
- ¼ teaspoon ginger, grated
- 1 garlic clove, minced

Directions:

1. Put soy sauce in a pan, heat up over medium heat, add mirin, sugar, lime and orange juice, pepper flakes, ginger and garlic, stir well, bring to a boil and take off heat.

2. Transfer half of the marinade to a bowl, add halibut, toss to coat and leave aside in the fridge for 30 minutes.

3. Transfer halibut to your air fryer and cook at 390 degrees F for 10 minutes, flipping once.

4. Divide halibut steaks on plates, drizzle the rest of the marinade all over and serve hot.

5. Enjoy!

Nutrition Values: calories 286, fat 5, fiber 12, carbs 14, protein 23

Cod and Vinaigrette

Preparation time: 10 minutes

Cooking time: 15 minutes

Servings: 4

Ingredients:

- 4 cod fillets, skinless and boneless
- 12 cherry tomatoes, halved
- 8 black olives, pitted and roughly chopped
- 2 tablespoons lemon juice
- Salt and black pepper to the taste
- 2 tablespoons olive oil
- Cooking spray
- 1 bunch basil, chopped

Directions:

1. Season cod with salt and pepper to the taste, place in your air fryer's basket and cook at 360 degrees F for 10 minutes, flipping after 5 minutes.

2. Meanwhile, heat up a pan with the oil over medium heat, add tomatoes, olives and lemon juice, stir, bring to a simmer, add

basil, salt and pepper, stir well and take off heat.

3. Divide fish on plates and serve with the vinaigrette drizzled on top.

4. Enjoy!

Nutrition Values: calories 300, fat 5, fiber 8, carbs 12, protein 8

Shrimp and Crab Mix

Preparation time: 10 minutes

Cooking time: 25 minutes

Servings: 4

Ingredients:

- ½ cup yellow onion, chopped
- 1 cup green bell pepper, chopped
- 1 cup celery, chopped
- 1 pound shrimp, peeled and deveined
- 1 cup crabmeat, flaked
- 1 cup mayonnaise
- 1 teaspoon Worcestershire sauce
- Salt and black pepper to the taste
- 2 tablespoons breadcrumbs
- 1 tablespoon butter, melted
- 1 teaspoon sweet paprika

Directions:

1. In a bowl, mix shrimp with crab meat, bell pepper, onion, mayo, celery, salt, pepper and Worcestershire sauce, toss well and transfer to a pan that fits your air fryer.

2. Sprinkle bread crumbs and paprika, add melted butter, place in your air fryer and cook at 320 degrees F for 25 minutes, shaking halfway.

3. Divide among plates and serve right away.

4. Enjoy!

Nutrition Values: calories 200, fat 13, fiber 9, carbs 17, protein 19

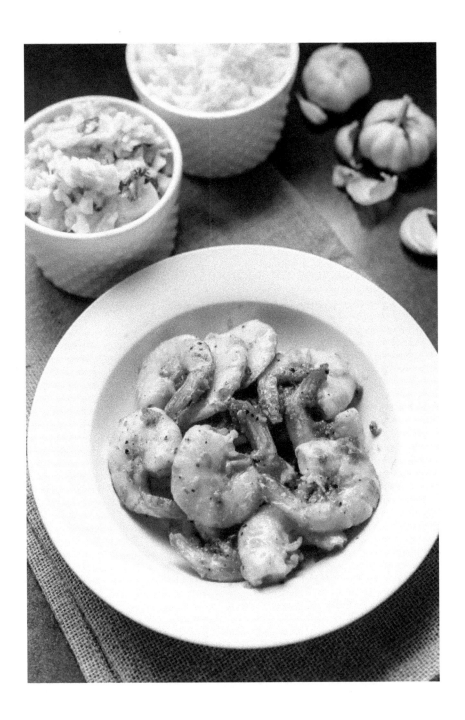

Seafood Casserole

Preparation time: 10 minutes

Cooking time: 40 minutes

Servings: 6

Ingredients:

- 6 tablespoons butter
- 2 ounces mushrooms, chopped
- 1 small green bell pepper, chopped
- 1 celery stalk, chopped
- 2 garlic cloves, minced
- 1 small yellow onion, chopped
- Salt and black pepper to the taste
- 4 tablespoons flour
- ½ cup white wine
- 1 and ½ cups milk
- ½ cup heavy cream
- 4 sea scallops, sliced
- 4 ounces haddock, skinless, boneless and cut into small pieces
- 4 ounces lobster meat, already cooked and cut into small pieces

- ½ teaspoon mustard powder

- 1 tablespoon lemon juice

- 1/3 cup bread crumbs

- Salt and black pepper to the taste

- 3 tablespoons cheddar cheese, grated

- A handful parsley, chopped

- 1 teaspoon sweet paprika

Directions:

1. Heat up a pan with 4 tablespoons butter over medium high heat, add bell pepper, mushrooms, celery, garlic, onion and wine, stir and cook for 10 minutes

2. Add flour, cream and milk, stir well and cook for 6 minutes.

3. Add lemon juice, salt, pepper, mustard powder, scallops, lobster meat and haddock, stir well, take off heat and transfer to a pan that fits your air fryer.

4. In a bowl, mix the rest of the butter with bread crumbs, paprika and cheese and sprinkle over seafood mix.

5. Transfer pan to your air fryer and cook at 360 degrees F for 16 minutes.

6. Divide among plates and serve with parsley sprinkled on top.

7. Enjoy!

Nutrition Values: calories 270, fat 32, fiber 14, carbs 15, protein 23

Trout Fillet and Orange Sauce

Preparation time: 10 minutes

Cooking time: 10 minutes

Servings: 4

Ingredients:

- 4 trout fillets, skinless and boneless
- 4 spring onions, chopped
- 1 tablespoon olive oil
- 1 tablespoon ginger, minced
- Salt and black pepper to the taste
- Juice and zest from 1 orange

Directions:

1. Season trout fillets with salt, pepper, rub them with the olive oil, place in a pan that fits your air fryer, add ginger, green onions, orange zest and juice, toss well, place in your air fryer and cook at 360 degrees F for 10 minutes.

2. Divide fish and sauce on plates and serve right away.

3. Enjoy!

Nutrition Values: calories 239, fat 10, fiber 7, carbs 18, protein 23

Cod Fillets and Peas

Preparation time: 10 minutes

Cooking time: 10 minutes

Servings: 4

Ingredients:

- 4 cod fillets, boneless
- 2 tablespoons parsley, chopped
- 2 cups peas
- 4 tablespoons wine
- ½ teaspoon oregano, dried
- ½ teaspoon sweet paprika
- 2 garlic cloves, minced
- Salt and pepper to the taste

Directions:

1. In your food processor mix garlic with parsley, salt, pepper, oregano, paprika and wine and blend well.

2. Rub fish with half of this mix, place in your air fryer and cook at 360 degrees F for 10 minutes.

3. Meanwhile, put peas in a pot, add water to cover, add salt, bring to a boil over medium high heat, cook for 10 minutes, drain and divide among plates.

4. Also divide fish on plates, spread the rest of the herb dressing all over and serve.

5. Enjoy!

Nutrition Values: calories 261, fat 8, fiber 12, carbs 20, protein 22

Crispylicious Crab Cakes

Servings: 2

Cooking Time: 10 minutes

Ingredients:

- 2 large eggs
- 1 teaspoon Dijon mustard
- 1 teaspoon Worcestershire sauce
- 1 ½ teaspoon old bay seasoning
- Salt and pepper to taste
- ¼ cup chopped green onion
- 1-pound lump crab meat
- ½ cup panko

Directions:

1. Preheat the air fryer at 3900F.

2. Place the grill pan accessory in the air fryer.

3. In a mixing bowl, combine all Ingredients: until everything is well-incorporated.

4. Use your hands to form small patties of crab cakes.

5. Place on the grill pan and cook for 10 minutes.

6. Flip the crab cakes halfway through the cooking time for even browning.

Nutrition Values:

Calories: 129; Carbs: 4.3g; Protein: 16.2g; Fat: 5.1g

Coconut Shrimps with Pina Colada Dip

Servings: 4

Cooking Time: 6 minutes

Ingredients:

- 1 ½ pounds jumbo shrimps, peeled and deveined
- ½ cup cornstarch
- 2/3 cup coconut milk
- 2 tablespoons honey
- 1 cup shredded coconut flakes
- ¾ cups panko bread crumbs
- 1/3 cup light coconut milk
- 1/3 cup non-fat Greek yogurt
- ¼ cup pineapple chunks, drained
- Salt and pepper to taste
- Toasted coconut meat for garnish

Directions:

1. Preheat the air fryer at 3900F.

2. Place the shrimps and cornstarch in a Ziploc bag and give a good shake.

3. In a bowl, stir in coconut milk and honey. Set aside.

4. In another bowl, mix the coconut flakes and bread crumbs. Set aside.

5. Dip the shrimps in the milk mixture then dredge in the bread crumbs.

6. Place in the double layer rack and cook for 6 minutes.

7. Meanwhile, combine the rest of the Ingredients: to create the dipping sauce.

Nutrition Values:

Calories: 493; Carbs: 21.4g; Protein: 38.9g; Fat: 27.9g

Alaskan Cod Fish with Apple Slaw

Servings: 3

Cooking Time: 15 minutes

Ingredients:

- 1 ½ pounds frozen Alaskan cod
- 1 tablespoon vegetable oil
- 1 box whole wheat panko bread crumbs
- 1 granny smith apple, julienned
- 2 cups Napa cabbage, shredded
- ½ red onion, diced
- ¼ cup mayonnaise
- 1 teaspoon paprika
- Salt and pepper to taste

Directions:

1. Preheat the air fryer at 3900F.

2. Place the grill pan accessory in the air fryer.

3. Brush the fish with oil and dredge in the breadcrumbs.

4. Place the fish on the grill pan and cook for 15 minutes. Make sure to flip the fish halfway through the cooking time.

5. Meanwhile, prepare the slaw by mixing the remaining Ingredients: in a bowl.

6. Serve the fish with the slaw.

Nutrition Values:

Calories: 316; Carbs: 13.5g; Protein: 37.8g; Fat: 12.2g

Beer Battered Air Fried Fish

Servings: 2

Cooking Time: 15 minutes

Ingredients:

- 2 cod fillets
- 2 eggs, beaten
- 1 ¼ cup lager beer
- ½ cup all-purpose flour
- ¾ teaspoon baking powder
- Salt and pepper to taste

Directions:

1. Preheat the air fryer at 3900F.
2. Pat the fish fillets dry then set aside.
3. In a bowl, combine the rest of the Ingredients: to create a batter.
4. Dip the fillets on the batter and place on the double layer rack.
5. Cook for 15 minutes.

Nutrition Values:

Calories: 229; Carbs: 33.2g; Protein: 31.1g; Fat: 10.2g

Blackened Shrimps in Air Fryer

Servings: 4

Cooking Time: 6 minutes

Ingredients:

- 20 jumbo shrimps, peeled and deveined
- 2 tablespoons coconut oil
- 2 teaspoons cilantro
- 2 teaspoons smoked paprika
- 2 teaspoons onion powder
- 1 teaspoon cumin
- 1 teaspoon salt
- 1 teaspoon thyme
- 1 teaspoon oregano
- ¼ teaspoon cayenne pepper
- ¼ teaspoon red chili flakes

Directions:

1. Preheat the air fryer at 3900F.

2. Season the shrimps with all the Ingredients.

3. Place the seasoned shrimps in the double layer rack.

4. Cook for 6 minutes.

Nutrition Values:

Calories: 220; Carbs: 2.5g; Protein: 34.2g; Fat: 8.1g

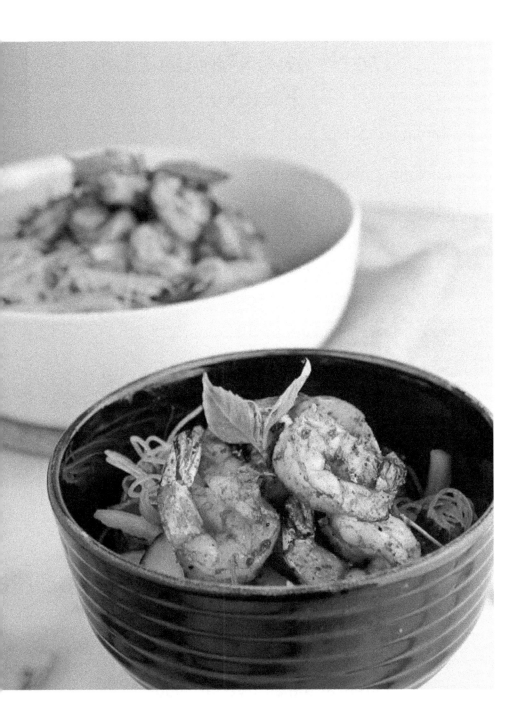

Herb and Garlic Fish Fingers

Servings: 1

Cooking Time: 10 minutes

Ingredients:

- ½ pound fish, cut into fingers
- ½ teaspoon salt
- 2 tablespoons lemon juice
- ½ teaspoon turmeric powder
- ½ teaspoon red chili flakes
- 2 teaspoons garlic powder
- ½ teaspoon crushed black pepper
- 1 teaspoon ginger garlic paste
- 2 teaspoons corn flour
- 2 eggs, beaten
- ¼ teaspoon baking soda
- 1 cup bread crumbs
- Oil for brushing

Directions:

1. Preheat the air fryer at 3900F.

2. Season the fish fingers with salt, lemon juice, turmeric powder, chili flakes, garlic powder, black pepper, and garlic paste. Add the corn flour, eggs, and baking soda.

3. Dredge the seasoned fish in breadcrumbs and brush with cooking oil.

4. Place on the double layer rack.

5. Cook for 10 minutes.

Nutrition Values:

Calories: 773; Carbs: 32.7g; Protein: 64.9g; Fat: 42.5gUBSCRIBE TO WHISKAFFAIR

Crispy Cod Nuggets with Tartar Sauce

Servings: 3

Cooking Time: 10 minutes

Ingredients:

- 1 ½ pounds cod fillet
- Salt and pepper to taste
- ½ cup flour
- 1 egg, beaten
- 1 cup cracker crumbs
- 1 tablespoon vegetable oil
- ½ cup non-fat mayonnaise
- 1 teaspoon honey
- Zest from half of a lemon
- Juice from half a lemon
- ½ teaspoon Worcestershire sauce
- 1 tablespoon sweet pickle relish
- Salt and pepper to taste

Directions:

1. Preheat the air fryer at 3900F.

2. Season the cods with salt and pepper.

3. Dredge the fish on flour and dip in the beaten egg before dredging on the cracker crumbs. Brush with oil.

4. Place the fish on the double layer rack and cook for 10 minutes.

5. Meanwhile, prepare the sauce by mixing all ingredients in a bowl.

6. Serve the fish with the sauce.

Nutrition Values:

Calories: 470; Carbs: 25.4g; Protein: 42.9g; Fat: 21.8g

Garlic and Black Pepper Shrimp Grill

Servings: 2

Cooking Time: 6 minutes

Ingredients:

- 1 red chili, seeds removed
- 3 cloves of garlic, grated
- 1 tablespoon ground pepper
- 1 tablespoon fresh lime juice
- 1-pound large shrimps, peeled and deveined
- Salt to taste

Directions:

1. Preheat the air fryer at 3900F.

2. Place the grill pan accessory in the air fryer.

3. Grill the shrimps for 6 minutes.

Nutrition Values:

Calories:179 ; Carbs: 6.3g; Protein: 31.6g; Fat: 2.3g

Grilled Salmon with Cucumbers

Servings: 4

Cooking Time: 10 minutes

Ingredients:

- 4 6-ounces salmon fillets
- 1 teaspoon lemon zest
- Juice from 1 lemon, freshly squeezed
- 1 tablespoon fresh dill
- Salt and pepper to taste
- ½ cup mayonnaise
- ½ cup sour cream
- 2 cucumbers peeled and sliced

Directions:

1. Preheat the air fryer at 3900F.

2. Place the grill pan accessory in the air fryer.

3. Season the salmon fillets with lemon zest, lemon juice, dill, salt and pepper.

4. 10Grill the salmon for 10 minutes making sure to flip halfway through the cooking time.

5. 11Meanwhile, prepare the cucumber salad by mixing in a bowl the mayonnaise, sour cream and cucumber slices. Season with salt and pepper.

6. 12Serve the salmon with the cucumber salad.

Nutrition Values:

Calories: 409; Carbs: 5.9g; Protein: 38.4g; Fat: 25.1g

Shrimps, Zucchini, And Tomatoes on the Grill

Servings: 2

Cooking Time: 15 minutes

Ingredients:

- 10 jumbo shrimps, peeled and deveined
- Salt and pepper to taste
- 1 clove of garlic, minced
- 1 medium zucchini, sliced
- 1-pint cherry tomatoes
- ¼ cup feta cheese

Directions:

1. Preheat the air fryer at 3900F.

2. Place the grill pan accessory in the air fryer.

3. In a mixing bowl, season the shrimps with salt and pepper. Stir in the garlic, zucchini, and tomatoes.

4. Place on the grill pan and cook for 15 minutes.

5. 10Once cooked, transfer to a bowl and sprinkle with feta cheese.

Nutrition Values:

Calories: 257; Carbs:4.2 g; Protein: 48.9g; Fat: 5.3g

Grilled Halibut with Tomatoes and Hearts of Palm

Servings: 4

Cooking Time: 15 minutes

Ingredients:

- 4 halibut fillets
- Juice from 1 lemon
- Salt and pepper to taste
- 2 tablespoons oil
- ½ cup hearts of palm, rinse and drained
- 1 cup cherry tomatoes

Directions:

1. Preheat the air fryer at 3900F.

2. Place the grill pan accessory in the air fryer.

3. Season the halibut fillets with lemon juice, salt and pepper. Brush with oil.

4. 10Place the fish on the grill pan.

5. 11Arrange the hearts of palms and cherry tomatoes on the side and sprinkle with more salt and pepper.

6. 12Cook for 15 minutes.

Nutrition Values:

Calories: 208; Carbs: 7g; Protein: 21 g; Fat: 11g

Chat Masala Grilled Snapper

Servings: 5

Cooking Time: 25 minutes

Ingredients:

- 2 ½ pounds whole fish
- Salt to taste
- 1/3 cup chat masala
- 3 tablespoons fresh lime juice
- 5 tablespoons olive oil

Directions:

1. Preheat the air fryer at 3900F.

2. Place the grill pan accessory in the air fryer.

3. Season the fish with salt, chat masala and lime juice.

4. 10Brush with oil

5. 11Place the fish on a foil basket and place inside the grill.

6. 12Cook for 25 minutes.

Nutrition Values:

Calories:308 ; Carbs: 0.7g; Protein: 35.2g; Fat: 17.4g

One-Pan Shrimp and Chorizo Mix Grill

Servings: 4

Cooking Time: 15 minutes

Ingredients:

- 1 ½ pounds large shrimps, peeled and deveined
- Salt and pepper to taste
- 6 links fresh chorizo sausage
- 2 bunches asparagus spears, trimmed
- Lime wedges

Directions:

1. Preheat the air fryer at 3900F.

2. Place the grill pan accessory in the air fryer.

3. 10Season the shrimps with salt and pepper to taste. Set aside.

4. 11Place the chorizo on the grill pan and the sausage.

5. 12Place the asparagus on top.

6. 13Grill for 15 minutes.

7. 14Serve with lime wedges.

Nutrition Values:

Calories:124 ; Carbs: 9.4g; Protein: 8.2g; Fat: 7.1g

Grilled Tasty Scallops

Servings: 2

Cooking Time: 10 minutes

Ingredients:

- 1-pound sea scallops, cleaned and patted dry
- Salt and pepper to taste
- 3 dried chilies
- 2 tablespoon dried thyme
- 1 tablespoon dried oregano
- 1 tablespoon ground coriander
- 1 tablespoon ground fennel
- 2 teaspoons chipotle pepper

Directions:

1. Preheat the air fryer at 3900F.
2. Place the grill pan accessory in the air fryer.
3. Mix all Ingredients: in a bowl.
4. Dump the scallops on the grill pan and cook for 10 minutes.

Nutrition Values:

Calories:291 ; Carbs: 20.7g; Protein: 48.6g; Fat: 2.5g

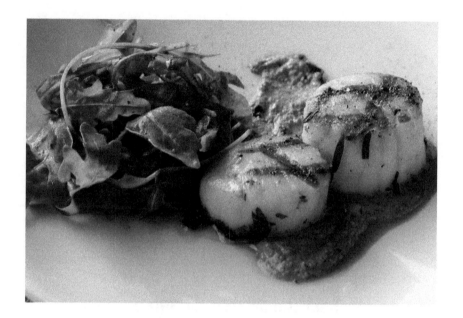

Clam with Lemons on the Grill

Servings: 6

Cooking Time: 6 minutes

Ingredients:

- 4 pounds littleneck clams
- Salt and pepper to taste
- 1 clove of garlic, minced
- ½ cup parsley, chopped
- 1 teaspoon crushed red pepper flakes
- 5 tablespoons olive oil
- 1 loaf crusty bread, halved
- ½ cup parmesan cheese, grated

Directions:

1. Preheat the air fryer at 3900F.

2. Place the grill pan accessory in the air fryer.

3. 10Place the clams on the grill pan and cook for 6 minutes.

4. 11Once the clams have opened, take them out and extract the meat.

5. 12Transfer the meat into a bowl and season with salt and pepper.

6. 13Stir in the garlic, parsley, red pepper flakes, and olive oil.

7. 14Serve on top of bread and sprinkle with parmesan cheese.

Nutrition Values:

Calories: 341; Carbs: 26g; Protein:48.3g; Fat: 17.2g

Salmon Steak Grilled with Cilantro Garlic Sauce

Servings: 2

Cooking Time: 15 minutes

Ingredients:

- 2 salmon steaks
- Salt and pepper to taste
- 2 tablespoons vegetable oil
- 2 cloves of garlic, minced
- 1 cup cilantro leaves
- ½ cup Greek yogurt
- 1 teaspoon honey

Directions:

1. Preheat the air fryer at 3900F.

2. Place the grill pan accessory in the air fryer.

3. Season the salmon steaks with salt and pepper. Brush with oil.

4. Grill for 15 minutes and make sure to flip halfway through the cooking time.

5. In a food processor, mix the garlic, cilantro leaves, yogurt and honey. Season with salt and pepper to taste. Pulse until smooth.

6. Serve the salmon steaks with the cilantro sauce.

Nutrition Values:

Calories: 485; Carbs: 6.3g; Protein: 47.6g; Fat: 29.9g

Tasty Grilled Red Mullet

Servings: 8

Cooking Time: 15 minutes

Ingredients:

- 8 whole red mullets, gutted and scales removed
- Salt and pepper to taste
- Juice from 1 lemon
- 1 tablespoon olive oil

Directions:

1. Preheat the air fryer at 3900F.

2. Place the grill pan accessory in the air fryer.

3. Season the red mullet with salt, pepper, and lemon juice.

4. Brush with olive oil.

5. Grill for 15 minutes.

Nutrition Values:

Calories: 152; Carbs: 0.9g; Protein: 23.1g; Fat: 6.2g

Chargrilled Halibut Niçoise With Vegetables

Servings: 6

Cooking Time: 15 minutes

Ingredients:

- 1 ½ pounds halibut fillets
- Salt and pepper to taste
- 2 tablespoons olive oil
- 2 pounds mixed vegetables
- 4 cups torn lettuce leaves
- 1 cup cherry tomatoes, halved
- 4 large hard-boiled eggs, peeled and sliced

Directions:

1. Preheat the air fryer at 3900F.

2. Place the grill pan accessory in the air fryer.

3. Rub the halibut with salt and pepper. Brush the fish with oil.

4. Place on the grill.

5. Surround the fish fillet with the mixed vegetables and cook for 15 minutes.

6. Assemble the salad by serving the fish fillet with grilled mixed vegetables, lettuce, cherry tomatoes, and hard-boiled eggs.

Nutrition Values:

Calories: 312; Carbs:16.8 g; Protein: 19.8g; Fat: 18.3g

Spiced Salmon Kebabs

Servings: 3

Cooking Time: 15 minutes

Ingredients:

- 2 tablespoons chopped fresh oregano
- 2 teaspoons sesame seeds
- 1 teaspoon ground cumin
- Salt and pepper to taste
- 1 ½ pounds salmon fillets
- 2 tablespoons olive oil
- 2 lemons, sliced into rounds

Directions:

1. Preheat the air fryer at 3900F.

2. Place the grill pan accessory in the air fryer.

3. Create the dry rub by combining the oregano, sesame seeds, cumin, salt and pepper.

4. Rub the salmon fillets with the dry rub and brush with oil.

5. Grill the salmon for 15 minutes.

6. Serve with lemon slices once cooked.

Nutrition Values:

Calories per serving 447 ; Carbs: 4.1g; Protein:47.6 g; Fat:26.6 g

Roasted Tuna on Linguine

Servings: 2

Cooking Time: 20 minutes

Ingredients:

- 1-pound fresh tuna fillets
- Salt and pepper to taste
- 1 tablespoon olive oil
- 12 ounces linguine, cooked according to package Directions:
- 2 cups parsley leaves, chopped
- 1 tablespoon capers, chopped
- Juice from 1 lemon

Directions:

1. Preheat the air fryer at 3900F.
2. Place the grill pan accessory in the air fryer.
3. Season the tuna with salt and pepper. Brush with oil.
4. Grill for 20 minutes.
5. Once the tuna is cooked, shred using forks and place on top of cooked linguine. Add

parsley and capers. Season with salt and pepper and add lemon juice.

Nutrition Values:

Calories: 520; Carbs: 60.6g; Protein: 47.7g; Fat: 9.6g

Chili Lime Clams with Tomatoes

Servings: 3

Cooking Time: 15 minutes

Ingredients:

- 25 littleneck clams
- 1 tablespoon fresh lime juice
- Salt and pepper to taste
- 6 tablespoons unsalted butter
- 4 cloves of garlic, minced
- ½ cup tomatoes, chopped
- ½ cup basil leaves

Directions:

1. Preheat the air fryer at 3900F.
2. Place the grill pan accessory in the air fryer.
3. On a large foil, place all ingredients. Fold over the foil and close by crimping the edges.
4. Place on the grill pan and cook for 15 minutes.
5. Serve with bread.

Nutrition Values:

Calories: 163; Carbs: 4.1g; Protein: 1.7g; Fat: 15.5g

Air Fryer Garlicky-Grilled Turbot

Servings: 2

Cooking Time: 20 minutes

Ingredients:

- 2 whole turbot, scaled and head removed
- Salt and pepper to taste
- 1 clove of garlic, minced
- ½ cup chopped celery leaves
- 2 tablespoons olive oil

Directions:

1. Preheat the air fryer at 3900F.

2. Place the grill pan accessory in the air fryer.

3. Season the turbot with salt, pepper, garlic, and celery leaves.

4. Brush with oil.

5. Place on the grill pan and cook for 20 minutes until the fish becomes flaky.

Nutrition Values:

Calories: 269; Carbs: 3.3g; Protein: 66.2g; Fat: 25.6g

Broiled Spiced-Lemon Squid

Servings: 4

Cooking Time: 15 minutes

Ingredients:

- 2 pounds squid, gutted and cleaned
- Salt and pepper to taste
- 1 tablespoon fresh lemon juice
- 5 cloves of garlic
- ½ cup tomatoes, chopped
- ½ cup green onions, chopped
- 2 tablespoons olive oil

Directions:

1. Preheat the air fryer at 3900F.

2. Place the grill pan accessory in the air fryer.

3. Season the squid with salt, pepper, and lemon juice.

4. Stuff the cavity with garlic, tomatoes, and onions.

5. Brush the squid with olive oil.

6. Place on the grill pan and cook for 15 minutes.

7. Halfway through the cooking time, flip the squid.

Nutrition Values:

Calories: 277; Carbs: 10.7g; Protein: 36g; Fat: 10g

Tuna Grill with Ginger Sauce

Servings: 3

Cooking Time: 20 minutes

Ingredients:

- 1 ½ pounds tuna, thick slices
- 2 tablespoons rice vinegar
- 2 tablespoons grated fresh ginger
- 2 tablespoons peanut oil
- 2 tablespoons soy sauce
- 2 tablespoons honey
- 1 serrano chili, seeded and minced

Directions:

1. Place all ingredients in a Ziploc bag.
2. Allow to marinate in the fridge for at least 2 hours.
3. Preheat the air fryer at 3900F.
4. Place the grill pan accessory in the air fryer.
5. Grill the fish for 15 to 20 minutes.
6. Flip the fish halfway through the cooking time.

7. Meanwhile, pour the marinade in a saucepan and allow to simmer for 10 minutes until the sauce thickens.

8. Brush the tuna with the sauce before serving.

Nutrition Values:

Calories: 357; Carbs:14.8 g; Protein: 44.9g; Fat: 13.1g

Char-Grilled Spicy Halibut

Servings: 6

Cooking Time: 20 minutes

Ingredients:

- 3 pounds halibut fillet, skin removed
- Salt and pepper to taste
- 4 tablespoons dry white wine
- 4 tablespoons olive oil
- 2 cloves of garlic, minced
- 1 tablespoon chili powder

Directions:

1. Place all ingredients in a Ziploc bag.
2. Allow to marinate in the fridge for at least 2 hours.
3. Preheat the air fryer at 3900F.
4. Place the grill pan accessory in the air fryer.
5. Grill the fish for 20 minutes making sure to flip every 5 minutes.

Nutrition Values:

Calories: 385; Carbs: 1.7g; Protein: 33g; Fat: 40.6g

Roasted Swordfish with Charred Leeks

Servings: 4

Cooking Time: 20 minutes

Ingredients:

- 4 swordfish steaks
- Salt and pepper to taste
- 3 tablespoons lime juice
- 2 tablespoons olive oil
- 4 medium leeks, cut into an inch long

Directions:

1. Preheat the air fryer at 3900F.
2. Place the grill pan accessory in the air fryer.
3. Season the swordfish with salt, pepper and lime juice.
4. Brush the fish with olive oil
5. Place fish fillets on grill pan and top with leeks.
6. Grill for 20 minutes.

Nutrition Values:

Calories: 611; Carbs: 14.6g; Protein: 48g; Fat: 40g

Chinese Stuffed Chicken Recipe

Preparation Time: 45 Minutes

Servings: 8

Ingredients:

- 1 whole chicken
- 10 wolfberries
- 2 red chilies; chopped
- 4 ginger slices
- 1 yam; cubed
- 1 tsp. soy sauce
- 3 tsp. sesame oil
- Salt and white pepper to the taste

Directions:

1. Season chicken with salt, pepper, rub with soy sauce and sesame oil and stuff with wolfberries, yam cubes, chilies and ginger.

2. Place in your air fryer, cook at 400 °F, for 20 minutes and then at 360 °F, for 15 minutes. Carve chicken, divide among plates and serve.

Nutrition Values: Calories: 320; Fat: 12; Fiber: 17; Carbs: 22; Protein: 12

Chicken and Asparagus Recipe

Preparation Time: 30 Minutes

Servings: 4

Ingredients:

- 8 chicken wings; halved
- 8 asparagus spears
- 1 tbsp. rosemary; chopped
- 1 tsp. cumin; ground
- Salt and black pepper to the taste

Directions:

1. Pat dry chicken wings, season with salt, pepper, cumin and rosemary, put them in your air fryer's basket and cook at 360 °F, for 20 minutes.

2. Meanwhile; heat up a pan over medium heat, add asparagus, add water to cover, steam for a few minutes; transfer to a bowl filled with ice water, drain and arrange on plates. Add chicken wings on the side and serve.

Nutrition Values: Calories: 270; Fat: 8; Fiber: 12; Carbs: 24; Protein: 22

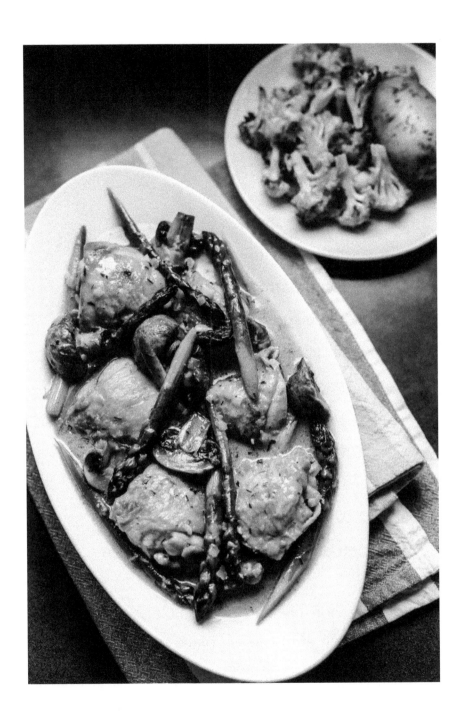

Italian Chicken Recipe

Preparation Time: 26 Minutes

Servings: 4

Ingredients:

- 5 chicken thighs
- 1 tbsp. olive oil
- 1/4 cup parmesan; grated
- 1/2 cup sun dried tomatoes
- 2 garlic cloves; minced
- 1 tbsp. thyme; chopped.
- 1/2 cup heavy cream
- 3/4 cup chicken stock
- 1 tsp. red pepper flakes; crushed
- 2 tbsp. basil; chopped
- Salt and black pepper to the taste

Directions:

1. Season chicken with salt and pepper, rub with half of the oil, place in your preheated air fryer at 350 °F and cook for 4 minutes.

2. Meanwhile; heat up a pan with the rest of the oil over medium high heat, add thyme garlic, pepper flakes, sun dried tomatoes, heavy cream, stock, parmesan, salt and pepper; stir, bring to a simmer, take off heat and transfer to a dish that fits your air fryer.

3. Add chicken thighs on top, introduce in your air fryer and cook at 320 °F, for 12 minutes. Divide among plates and serve with basil sprinkled on top.

Nutrition Values: Calories: 272; Fat: 9; Fiber: 12; Carbs: 37; Protein: 23

Chinese Chicken Wings Recipe

Preparation Time: 2 hours 15 Minutes

Servings: 6

Ingredients:

- 16 chicken wings
- 2 tbsp. honey
- 2 tbsp. soy sauce
- Salt and black pepper to the taste
- 1/4 tsp. white pepper
- 3 tbsp. lime juice

Directions:

1. In a bowl, mix honey with soy sauce, salt, black and white pepper and lime juice, whisk well, add chicken pieces, toss to coat and keep in the fridge for 2 hours.

2. Transfer chicken to your air fryer, cook at 370 °F, for 6 minutes on each side, increase heat to 400 °F and cook for 3 minutes more. Serve hot.

Nutrition Values: Calories: 372; Fat: 9; Fiber: 10; Carbs: 37; Protein: 24

Creamy Chicken, Peas and Rice

Preparation Time: 40 Minutes

Servings: 4

Ingredients:

- 1 lb. chicken breasts; skinless, boneless and cut into quarters
- 1 cup white rice; already cooked
- 1 cup chicken stock
- 1/4 cup parsley; chopped.
- 2 cups peas; frozen
- 1 ½ cups parmesan; grated
- 1 tbsp. olive oil
- 3 garlic cloves; minced
- 1 yellow onion; chopped
- 1/2 cup white wine
- 1/4 cup heavy cream
- Salt and black pepper to the taste

Directions:

1. Season chicken breasts with salt and pepper, drizzle half of the oil over them, rub

well, put in your air fryer's basket and cook them at 360 °F, for 6 minutes.

2. Heat up a pan with the rest of the oil over medium high heat, add garlic, onion, wine, stock, salt, pepper and heavy cream; stir, bring to a simmer and cook for 9 minutes.

3. Transfer chicken breasts to a heat proof dish that fits your air fryer, add peas, rice and cream mix over them, toss, sprinkle parmesan and parsley all over, place in your air fryer and cook at 420 °F, for 10 minutes. Divide among plates and serve hot.

Nutrition Values: Calories: 313; Fat: 12; Fiber: 14; Carbs: 27; Protein: 44

Chicken and Green Onions Sauce Recipe

Preparation Time: 26 Minutes

Servings: 4

Ingredients:

- 10 green onions; roughly chopped.
- 1-inch piece ginger root; chopped
- 4 garlic cloves; minced
- 2 tbsp. fish sauce
- 3 tbsp. soy sauce
- 1 tsp. Chinese five spice
- 10 chicken drumsticks
- 1 cup coconut milk
- 1 tsp. butter; melted
- 1/4 cup cilantro; chopped.
- 1 tbsp. lime juice
- Salt and black pepper to the taste

Directions:

1. In your food processor, mix green onions with ginger, garlic, soy sauce, fish sauce,

five spice, salt, pepper, butter and coconut milk and pulse well.

2. In a bowl, mix chicken with green onions mix; toss well, transfer everything to a pan that fits your air fryer and cook at 370 °F, for 16 minutes; shaking the fryer once. Divide among plates, sprinkle cilantro on top, drizzle lime juice and serve with a side salad.

Nutrition Values: Calories: 321; Fat: 12; Fiber: 12; Carbs: 22; Protein: 20

Chicken Cacciatore Recipe

Preparation Time: 30 Minutes

Servings: 4

Ingredients:

- 8 chicken drumsticks; bone-in
- 1/2 cup black olives; pitted and sliced
- 1 bay leaf
- 1 tsp. garlic powder
- 1 yellow onion; chopped
- 28 oz. canned tomatoes and juice; crushed
- 1 tsp. oregano; dried
- Salt and black pepper to the taste

Directions:

1. In a heat proof dish that fits your air fryer, mix chicken with salt, pepper, garlic powder, bay leaf, onion, tomatoes and juice, oregano and olives; toss, introduce in your preheated air fryer and cook at 365 °F, for 20 minutes. Divide among plates and serve.

Nutrition Values: Calories: 300; Fat: 12; Fiber: 8; Carbs: 20; Protein: 24

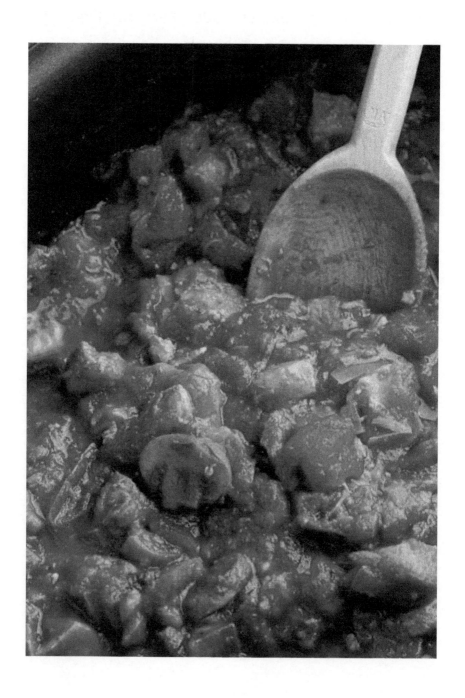

Herbed Chicken Recipe

Preparation Time: 70 Minutes

Servings: 4

Ingredients:

- 1 whole chicken
- 1 tsp. garlic powder
- 1 tsp. onion powder
- 1/2 tsp. thyme; dried
- 1 tsp. rosemary; dried
- 1 tbsp. lemon juice
- 2 tbsp. olive oil
- Salt and black pepper to the taste

Directions:

1. Season chicken with salt and pepper, rub with thyme, rosemary, garlic powder and onion powder, rub with lemon juice and olive oil and leave aside for 30 minutes.

2. Put chicken in your air fryer and cook at 360 °F, for 20 minutes on each side. Leave chicken aside to cool down, carve and serve.

Nutrition Values: Calories: 390; Fat: 10; Fiber: 5; Carbs: 22; Protein: 20

Air Fried Chicken with Honey and Lemon

Preparation Time: 100 min

Servings: 6

Nutrition Values: Calories: 342; Carbs: 68g; Fat: 28g; Protein: 33g

Ingredients

The Stuffing:

- 1 whole chicken, 3 lb
- 2 red and peeled onions
- 2 tbsp olive oil
- 2 apricots
- 1 zucchini
- 1 apple
- 2 cloves finely chopped garlic
- Fresh chopped thyme
- Salt and pepper

The Marinade:

- 5 oz honey

- juice from 1 lemon
- 2 tbsp olive oil
- Salt and pepper

Directions

1. For the stuffing, chop all ingredients into tiny pieces. Transfer to a large bowl and add the olive oil. Season with salt and black pepper. Fill the cavity of the chicken with the stuffing, without packing it tightly.

2. Place the chicken in the Air Fryer and cook for 35 minutes at 340 F. Warm the honey and the lemon juice in a large pan; season with salt and pepper. Reduce the temperature of the Air Fryer to 320 F.

3. Brush the chicken with some of the honey-lemon marinade and return it to the fryer. Cook for another 70 minutes; brush the chicken every 20-25 minutes with the marinade. Garnish with parsley, and serve with potatoes.

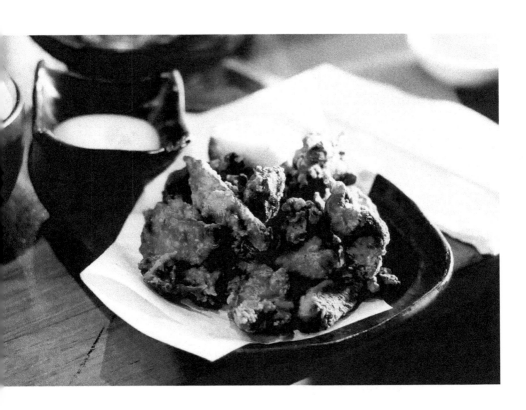

Spicy Honey Orange Chicken

Preparation Time: 20 min

Servings: 4

Nutrition Values: Calories: 246; Carbs: 21g; Fat: 6g; Protein: 25g

Ingredients

- 1 ½ pounds chicken breast, washed and sliced
- Parsley to taste
- 1 cup coconut, shredded
- ¾ cup breadcrumbs
- 2 whole eggs, beaten
- ½ cup flour
- ½ tsp pepper
- Salt to taste
- ½ cup orange marmalade
- 1 tbsp red pepper flakes
- ¼ cup honey
- 3 tbsp dijon mustard

Directions

1. Preheat your Air Fryer to 400 F. In a mixing bowl, combine coconut, flour, salt, parsley and pepper. In another bowl, add the beaten eggs. Place breadcrumbs in a third bowl. Dredge chicken in egg mix, flour and finally in the breadcrumbs. Place the chicken in the Air Fryer cooking basket and bake for 15 minutes.

2. In a separate bowl, mix honey, orange marmalade, mustard and pepper flakes. Cover chicken with marmalade mixture and fry for 5 more minutes. Enjoy!

Crunchy Chicken Fingers

Preparation Time: 8 min

Servings: 2

Nutrition Values: Calories: 253; Carbs: 31g; Fat: 18g; Protein: 28g

Ingredients

- 2 medium-sized chicken breasts, cut in stripes
- 3 tbsp parmesan cheese
- ¼ tbsp fresh chives, chopped
- ⅓ cup breadcrumbs
- 1 egg white
- 2 tbsp plum sauce, optional
- ½ tbsp fresh thyme, chopped
- ½ tbsp black pepper
- 1 tbsp water

Directions

1. Preheat the Air Fryer to 360 F. Mix the chives, parmesan, thyme, pepper and breadcrumbs. In another bowl, whisk the egg white and mix with the water. Dip the

chicken strips into the egg mixture and the breadcrumb mixture. Place the strips in the air fryer basket and cook for 10 minutes. Serve with plum sauce.

Mustard and Maple Turkey Breast

Preparation Time: 1 hr

Servings: 6

Nutrition Values: Calories: 529; Carbs: 77g; Fat: 20g; Protein: 13g

Ingredients

- 5 lb of whole turkey breast
- ¼ cup maple syrup
- 2 tbsp dijon mustard
- ½ tbsp smoked paprika
- 1 tbsp thyme
- 2 tbsp olive oil
- ½ tbsp sage
- ½ tbsp salt and black pepper
- 1 tbsp butter, melted

Directions

1. Preheat the Air fryer to 350 F and brush the turkey with the olive oil. Combine all herbs and seasoning, in a small bowl, and rub the turkey with the mixture. Air fry the turkey

for 25 minutes. Flip the turkey on its side and continue to cook for 12 more minutes.

2. Now, turn on the opposite side, and again, cook for an additional 12 minutes. Whisk the butter, maple and mustard together in a small bowl. When done, brush the glaze all over the turkey. Return to the air fryer and cook for 5 more minutes, until nice and crispy.

Chicken Breasts with Tarragon

Preparation Time: 15 min

Servings: 3

Nutrition Values: Calories: 493; Carbs: 36.5g; Fat: 11g; Protein: 57.5g

Ingredients

- 1 boneless and skinless chicken breast
- ½ tbsp butter
- ¼ tbsp kosher salt
- ¼ cup dried tarragon
- ¼ tbsp black and fresh ground pepper

Directions

1. Preheat the Air Fryer to 380 F and place each chicken breast on a 12x12 inches foil wrap. Top the chicken with tarragon and butter; season with salt and pepper to taste. Wrap the foil around the chicken breast in a loose way to create a flow of air. Cook the in the Air Fryer for 15 minutes. Carefully unwrap the chicken and serve.

Cajun Chicken Tenders

Preparation Time: 25 min

Servings: 4

Nutrition Values: Calories: 253; Carbs: 16g; Fat: 11g; Protein: 23.5g

Ingredients

- 3 lb chicken breast cut into slices
- 3 eggs
- 2 ¼ cup flour, divided
- 1 tbsp olive oil
- ½ tbsp plus
- ½ tbsp garlic powder, divided
- 1 tbsp salt
- 3 tbsp cajun seasoning, divided
- ¼ cup milk

Directions

1. Season the chicken with salt, pepper, ½ tbsp garlic powder and 2 tbsp Cajun seasoning.

2. Combine 2 cups flour, the rest of the Cajun seasoning and the rest of the garlic powder,

99

in a bowl. In another bowl, whisk the eggs, milk, olive oil, and quarter cup flour. Preheat the Air fryer to 370 F.

3. Line a baking sheet with parchment paper. Dip the chicken into the egg mixture first, and then into the flour mixture. Arrange on the sheet. If there isn't enough room, work in two batches. Cook for 12 to 15 minutes.

Chicken with Cashew Nuts

Preparation Time: 30 min

Servings: 4

Nutrition Values: Calories: 425; Carbs: 25g; Fat: 35g; Protein: 53g

Ingredients

- 1 lb chicken cubes
- 2 tbsp soy sauce
- 1 tbsp corn flour
- 2 ½ onion cubes
- 1 carrot, chopped
- ⅓ cup cashew nuts, fried
- 1 capsicum, cut
- 2 tbsp garlic, crushed
- Salt and white pepper

Directions

1. Marinate the chicken cubes with ½ tbsp of white pepper, ½ tsp salt, 2 tbsp soya sauce, and add 1 tbsp corn flour.

2. Set aside for 25 minutes. Preheat the Air Fryer to 380 F and transfer the marinated

chicken. Add the garlic, the onion, the capsicum, and the carrot; fry for 5-6 minutes. Roll it in the cashew nuts before serving.

Crunchy Coconut Chicken

Preparation Time: 22 min

Servings: 4

Nutrition Values: Calories: 651; Carbs: 21.6g; Fat: 47g; Protein: 66g

Ingredients

- 3 ½ cups coconut flakes
- 4 chicken breasts cut into strips
- ½ cup cornstarch
- ¼ tsp pepper
- ¼ tsp salt
- 3 eggs, beaten

Directions

1. Preheat the Air fryer to 350 F. Mix salt, pepper, and cornstarch in a small bowl. Line a baking sheet with parchment paper. Dip the chicken first in the cornstarch, then into the eggs, and finally, coat with coconut flakes. Arrange on the sheet and cook for 8 minutes. Flip the chicken over, and cook for 8 more minutes, until crispy.

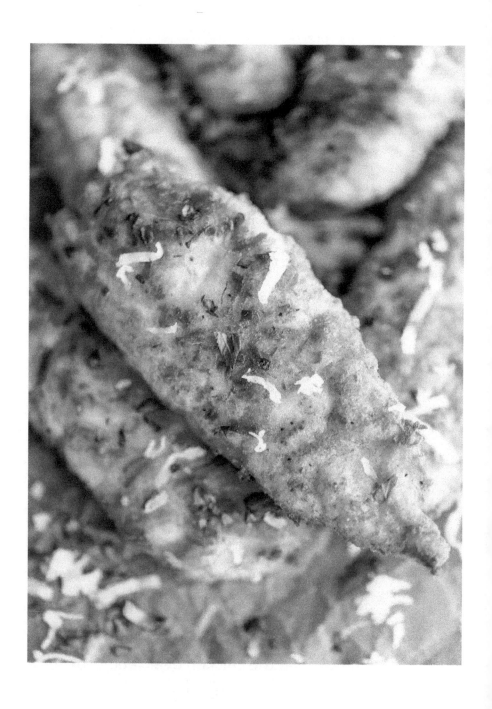

Air Fried Southern Drumsticks

Preparation Time: 50 min

Servings: 4

Nutrition Values: Calories: 197; Carbs: 5.2g; Fat: 6g; Protein: 29.2g

Ingredients

- 8 chicken drumsticks
- 2 tbsp oregano
- 2 tbsp thyme
- 2 oz oats
- ¼ cup milk
- ¼ steamed cauliflower florets
- 1 egg
- 1 tbsp ground cayenne
- Salt and pepper, to taste

Directions

1. Preheat the Air fryer to 350 F and season the drumsticks with salt and pepper; rub them with the milk. Place all the other ingredients, except the egg, in a food

processor. Process until smooth. Dip each drumstick in the egg first, and then in the oat mixture. Arrange half of them on a baking mat inside the air fryer. Cook for 20 minutes. Repeat with the other batch.

Fried Chicken Legs

Preparation Time: 50 min

Servings: 5

Nutrition Values: Calories: 288; Carbs: 15g; Fat: 11g; Protein: 35g

Ingredients

- 5 quarters chicken legs
- 2 lemons, halved
- 5 tbsp garlic powder
- 5 tbsp dried basil
- 5 tbsp oregano, dried
- ⅓ cup olive oil
- Salt and black pepper

Directions

1. Set the Air Fryer to 350 F. Place the chicken in a large deep bowl. Brush the chicken legs with a tbsp of olive oil.

2. Sprinkle with the lemon juice and arrange in the Air Fryer. In another bowl, combine basil, oregano, garlic powder, salt and pepper. Sprinkle the seasoning mixture on

the chicken. Cook in the preheated Air Fryer for 50 minutes, shaking every 10-15 minutes.

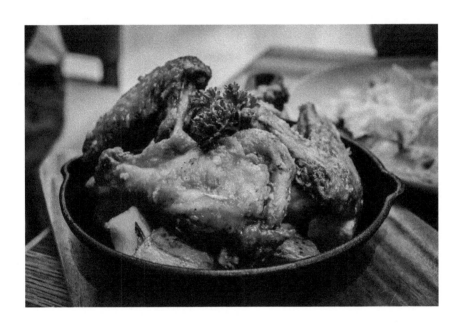

Lightning Source UK Ltd.
Milton Keynes UK
UKHW020801230621
386011UK00006B/34